SAXENDA Liraglutide Medical Usage

The ultimate guide to the anti-diabetic medication, weight loss drugs, dosage and side effects.

Dr Martins kimberly

Copyright © [2024] by Dr Martins Kimberly

All rights reserved. No part of this book may be reproduced or transmitted in any form or by any means, electronic or mechanical, including photocopying, recording, or by any information storage and retrieval system, without permission in writing from the author.

Disclaimer:

The information provided here is for general informational purposes only and is not intended to be a substitute for professional medical advice, diagnosis, or treatment. Always seek the advice of your physician or other qualified health provider with any questions you may have regarding a medical condition.

The content in this information does not constitute medical advice, and reliance on any information provided by this source is solely at your own risk. The author and publisher of this content are not medical professionals, and the content should not be considered as medical consultation.

Table of Contents

Introduction

1.1 Overview of Saxenda
1.2 Purpose of the Guide
Understanding Saxenda

2.1 What is Saxenda?
2.2 How Does Saxenda Work?
2.3 Approval and Safety
Indications and Usage

3.1 Who Can Benefit from Saxenda?
3.2 Medical Conditions and Considerations
Getting Started with Saxenda

4.1 Consultation with Healthcare Provider
4.2 Prescription and Dosage
4.3 Proper Injection Techniques
Saxenda and Weight Loss

5.1 Mechanisms of Weight Loss
5.2 Clinical Studies and Efficacy

5.3 Expected Results and Timelines
Nutritional Guidelines

6.1 Diet Recommendations
6.2 Meal Planning
6.3 Combining Saxenda with Healthy Eating
Incorporating Exercise

7.1 Importance of Physical Activity
7.2 Suitable Exercises
7.3 Creating a Fitness Routine
Managing Side Effects

8.1 Common Side Effects
8.2 When to Seek Medical Attention
8.3 Tips for Minimizing Discomfort
Success Stories

9.1 Real-Life Experiences
9.2 Inspirational Journeys
Maintaining Weight Loss

10.1 Post-Saxenda Strategies
10.2 Long-Term Lifestyle Changes
10.3 Preventing Weight Regain
FAQs about Saxenda

11.1 Addressing Common Queries
11.2 Clarifying Misconceptions
Conclusion

12.1 Recap of Key Points
12.2 Looking Ahead in Your Weight Loss Journey

Chapter 1

Introduction

1.1 Overview of Saxenda

Introduction to Saxenda

Saxenda, a brand name for liraglutide, is an FDA-approved prescription medication designed to aid in weight loss. It belongs to a class of drugs known as glucagon-like peptide-1 (GLP-1) receptor agonists. Originally developed for the treatment of type 2 diabetes, Saxenda has shown remarkable efficacy in promoting weight loss and is now prescribed specifically for that purpose.

Mechanism of Action

At the core of Saxenda's weight loss capabilities lies its ability to mimic the effects of GLP-1, a naturally occurring hormone in the body. GLP-1 plays a crucial role in regulating appetite and metabolism. Saxenda, as a synthetic GLP-1 analog, interacts with the receptors in the brain that control hunger and satiety, leading to reduced food intake and increased feelings of fullness.

FDA Approval and Safety

Saxenda received approval from the U.S. Food and Drug Administration (FDA) after rigorous clinical trials demonstrated its effectiveness and safety. It is important to note that Saxenda is not a standalone solution but is intended to be used in conjunction with a reduced-calorie diet and increased physical activity.

Target Population

Saxenda is typically prescribed for individuals with a body mass index (BMI) of 30 or higher, or for those with a BMI of 27 or higher with weight-related conditions such as hypertension, type 2 diabetes, or dyslipidemia. Before initiating Saxenda treatment, a thorough evaluation by a healthcare provider is crucial to ensure its suitability for the individual.

Duration of Treatment

The duration of Saxenda treatment varies and is often determined by the individual's response to the medication and their weight loss goals. It is essential to follow the prescribed dosage and any recommendations provided by the healthcare professional overseeing the treatment.

Notable Considerations
While Saxenda has shown significant success in aiding weight loss, it is not without considerations. Potential side effects, drug interactions, and contraindications exist and should be thoroughly discussed with a healthcare provider. Additionally, Saxenda is administered via subcutaneous injection, and proper technique and site rotation should be followed to optimize its effectiveness.

In essence, the overview of Saxenda sets the stage for a comprehensive understanding of this medication's role in weight loss. From its mechanism of action to safety considerations and target population, this section aims to provide a solid foundation for readers embarking on their journey with Saxenda.

1.2 Purpose of the Guide
Guiding Your Journey to Successful Weight Loss with Saxenda

Unveiling the Motivation

The purpose of this guide is to serve as a comprehensive companion for individuals embarking on a weight loss journey with Saxenda. In a world where obesity and its related health concerns are prevalent, Saxenda emerges as a promising tool. This guide aims to empower readers with the knowledge and insights needed to navigate this journey successfully.

Navigating the Complex Landscape

Weight loss is a complex and multifaceted endeavor. This guide recognizes the challenges individuals face and seeks to simplify the process by providing clear, evidence-based information. From understanding the intricacies of Saxenda's mechanism of action to practical tips for incorporating it into daily life, the guide aims to demystify the journey to a healthier weight.

Empowering Informed Decision-Making

Informed decision-making is at the core of successful weight loss. This guide aspires to empower readers with the knowledge needed to make informed choices about Saxenda. By offering a deep dive into its benefits, considerations, and potential outcomes, readers can approach their treatment with confidence and a clear understanding of what to expect.

Fostering a Holistic Approach

Weight loss is not solely about medications; it's a holistic journey that involves lifestyle changes, dietary modifications, and, often, a shift in mindset. This guide goes beyond the pharmaceutical aspects of Saxenda, delving into nutrition, exercise, and long-term strategies for maintaining weight loss. It encourages a holistic approach that extends beyond the prescription, emphasizing sustainable and health-centered habits.

Addressing Concerns and Questions

In the journey with Saxenda, questions and concerns are inevitable. The purpose of this guide is to preemptively address common queries, provide solutions to potential challenges, and offer guidance on maximizing the benefits of Saxenda. By doing so, it aims to foster a sense of assurance and support for individuals navigating the complexities of weight loss.

Building a Supportive Community

Embarking on a weight loss journey can feel isolating. The guide seeks to foster a sense of community among readers, acknowledging shared experiences and providing a platform for learning from the successes and challenges of others. It encourages readers to engage in their health journey actively and seek support when needed.

In summary, the purpose of this guide extends beyond being a mere informational resource. It aspires to be a companion, a mentor, and a source of empowerment for individuals incorporating Saxenda into their weight loss strategy. By unraveling the purpose, the guide sets the tone for a collaborative and informed approach to achieving and maintaining a healthier weight.

Chapter 2

Understanding Saxenda

2.1 What is Saxenda?
Unveiling the Nature of Saxenda
Introduction to Saxenda
Saxenda, a brand name for liraglutide, stands at the forefront of pharmaceutical interventions for weight loss. It belongs to the class of medications known as glucagon-like peptide-1 (GLP-1) receptor agonists. Originally developed as a treatment for type 2 diabetes, Saxenda has proven to be a valuable tool in promoting weight loss.

Synthetic GLP-1 Analog
At its core, Saxenda is a synthetic analog of GLP-1, a naturally occurring hormone in the body. GLP-1 plays a pivotal role in regulating glucose metabolism and appetite. By mimicking the actions of GLP-1, Saxenda influences the brain's appetite control centers, leading to reduced food intake and a sense of fullness.

FDA Approval for Weight Loss

Saxenda secured approval from the U.S. Food and Drug Administration (FDA) specifically for the purpose of weight loss. This distinction underscores its efficacy and safety in helping individuals achieve and maintain a healthier weight. It is important to note that Saxenda is not a standalone solution; it is intended to be part of a comprehensive weight loss plan that includes a reduced-calorie diet and increased physical activity.

Subcutaneous Injection Administration

Unlike traditional weight loss medications, Saxenda is administered via subcutaneous injection, typically in the abdomen, thigh, or upper arm. The injection is self-administered, and patients are usually provided with instructions on proper technique and rotation of injection sites to enhance effectiveness.

Target Population

Saxenda is primarily prescribed for individuals with a body mass index (BMI) of 30 or higher, or for those with a BMI of 27 or higher with weight-related comorbidities such as type 2 diabetes, hypertension, or dyslipidemia. This careful selection ensures that the medication is used in cases where the benefits outweigh potential risks.

Dual Role: Diabetes and Weight Loss
While initially developed for diabetes management, Saxenda's dual role in addressing both diabetes and promoting weight loss showcases its versatility. The guide will further explore how Saxenda's mechanism of action adapts to support weight loss goals, providing a unique synergy in managing metabolic health.

In essence, Saxenda emerges as a potent ally in the pursuit of weight loss, leveraging the body's natural mechanisms to regulate appetite and enhance satiety. This section lays the foundation for understanding the pharmacological nature of Saxenda and its distinct role in the realm of weight management.

2.2 How Does Saxenda Work?
Unraveling the Mechanisms Behind Saxenda's Efficacy
Mimicking the Actions of GLP-1

At the core of Saxenda's efficacy lies its ability to mimic the actions of a natural hormone in the body known as glucagon-like peptide-1 (GLP-1). GLP-1 plays a crucial role in regulating glucose metabolism and appetite. Saxenda, being a synthetic GLP-1 analog, engages with the GLP-1 receptors in the brain, particularly those that influence hunger and satiety.

Appetite Control Centers in the Brain
Saxenda's interaction with the appetite control centers in the brain leads to several key effects. Firstly, it reduces the sensation of hunger, making it easier for individuals to adhere to a reduced-calorie diet. Secondly, Saxenda enhances feelings of fullness, promoting satisfaction with smaller food portions and overall reduced food intake.

Slowing Gastric Emptying
Another significant mechanism of Saxenda is its impact on gastric emptying. It slows down the rate at which the stomach empties its contents into the intestines. This delay contributes to prolonged feelings of fullness after meals, aiding in portion control and reducing the likelihood of overeating.

Blood Glucose Regulation

While Saxenda's primary role is in weight management, its origins as a diabetes medication highlight its influence on blood glucose levels. Saxenda helps regulate blood glucose by modulating insulin secretion in response to meals. This dual benefit addresses not only weight concerns but also contributes to better metabolic control.

Complementary Lifestyle Changes

Saxenda is most effective when integrated into a comprehensive approach to weight loss. The guide emphasizes the importance of combining Saxenda with a reduced-calorie diet and increased physical activity. These lifestyle changes synergize with Saxenda's pharmacological effects, creating a holistic strategy for achieving and sustaining weight loss.

Gradual and Sustainable Results

Saxenda does not promise overnight transformations. Instead, it facilitates gradual and sustainable weight loss. The guide will delve into realistic expectations, helping individuals understand that Saxenda is a tool that, when used in conjunction with lifestyle changes, contributes to long-term success.

2.2

In summary, Saxenda's effectiveness in promoting weight loss stems from its ability to modulate key physiological processes related to appetite, satiety, and glucose metabolism. This section provides a detailed exploration of how Saxenda works at a molecular and physiological level, setting the stage for a nuanced understanding of its role in the weight loss journey.

2.3 Approval and Safety
Navigating the Regulatory Landscape
Rigorous FDA Approval

Saxenda's journey from a pharmaceutical concept to a weight loss solution involved rigorous scrutiny by the U.S. Food and Drug Administration (FDA). It received official approval, a testament to its demonstrated safety and efficacy in clinical trials. The FDA's stamp of approval signifies that Saxenda has met stringent standards, assuring users of its reliability and adherence to regulatory guidelines.

Safety Protocols and Clinical Trials

The approval process involved extensive clinical trials that evaluated Saxenda's safety profile across diverse populations. These trials assessed potential side effects, interactions with other medications, and the medication's overall impact on health. The guide will provide an overview of these safety protocols, ensuring readers understand the thorough testing Saxenda underwent before reaching the market.

Understanding Safety Measures

Healthcare Provider Oversight

Safety is paramount in Saxenda's usage, and the guide emphasizes the importance of seeking professional guidance. A licensed healthcare provider, after a comprehensive evaluation of an individual's health history and potential risk factors, prescribes Saxenda. This personalized approach ensures that the medication is used safely and effectively.

Addressing Potential Side Effects

No medication is without potential side effects, and Saxenda is no exception. The guide provides a detailed breakdown of common and rare side effects associated with Saxenda, empowering users with the knowledge to recognize and address any concerns promptly. Understanding the difference between expected and concerning side effects is vital for a safe and effective weight loss journey.

Monitoring and Adjusting Dosages
To enhance safety, healthcare providers may monitor individuals on Saxenda and adjust dosage as needed. The guide delves into the importance of regular check-ups, allowing healthcare professionals to assess progress, address concerns, and make any necessary adjustments to dosage or treatment plans.

User Responsibility and Education
Self-Administration Techniques
Saxenda is administered via subcutaneous injection, a process users can learn to perform independently. The guide provides step-by-step instructions on proper injection techniques, emphasizing the importance of adherence to guidelines for optimal results and safety.

Educating Users on Risks and Benefits

An informed user is an empowered one. The guide educates users on the potential risks and benefits of Saxenda, fostering a proactive approach to their health. By understanding the medication's safety profile, users can make informed decisions and communicate effectively with their healthcare providers.

2.3

This section sheds light on the robust approval process Saxenda underwent, assuring users of its safety and efficacy. It navigates the safety measures in place, from healthcare provider oversight to user responsibility, laying the groundwork for a secure and informed weight loss journey with Saxenda.

Chapter 3

Indications and Usage

3.1 Who Can Benefit from Saxenda?
Tailoring Saxenda to Specific Needs
Body Mass Index (BMI) Criteria
Saxenda is primarily prescribed for individuals with a specific body mass index (BMI) range. The guide introduces the concept of BMI and explains how it is calculated. Typically, Saxenda is considered for individuals with a BMI of 30 or higher. Alternatively, those with a BMI of 27 or higher may be eligible if they have weight-related conditions like type 2 diabetes, hypertension, or dyslipidemia.

Individualized Assessments
While BMI provides a general guideline, the guide underscores the importance of individualized assessments. Healthcare providers conduct thorough evaluations, taking into account an individual's overall health, medical history, and specific weight-related concerns. This personalized approach

ensures that Saxenda is prescribed to those who stand to benefit the most.

Identifying Potential Candidates
Individuals with Obesity-Related Conditions
Saxenda is particularly beneficial for individuals with obesity-related conditions such as type 2 diabetes, where weight management is crucial for overall health. The guide details how Saxenda's dual role in addressing weight and metabolic health makes it a valuable option for those navigating both challenges simultaneously.

Those Struggling with Traditional Weight Loss Methods
For individuals who have struggled with traditional weight loss methods, Saxenda offers a different approach. The guide explores scenarios where lifestyle changes alone may not have yielded the desired results, and Saxenda becomes a supportive tool in achieving sustainable weight loss.

Considerations and Precautions
Pre-existing Medical Conditions
The guide delves into considerations for individuals with pre-existing medical conditions, emphasizing

the importance of transparent communication with healthcare providers. Saxenda may not be suitable for everyone, and the guide educates users on potential contraindications and scenarios where alternative approaches might be considered.

Pregnancy and Lactation
Special considerations are outlined for individuals who are pregnant, planning to become pregnant, or breastfeeding. Saxenda's safety during pregnancy and lactation is discussed, and alternative strategies for weight management are explored for those in these specific life stages.

In summary, this section provides a nuanced understanding of who can benefit from Saxenda, emphasizing the role of BMI, individualized assessments, and specific scenarios where Saxenda becomes a valuable tool in the pursuit of weight loss. By addressing considerations and precautions, the guide ensures that readers approach Saxenda with a clear understanding of its applicability to their unique circumstances.

3.2 Medical Conditions and Considerations
Tailoring Saxenda to Individual Health

Comprehensive Health Evaluation

Before initiating Saxenda, a comprehensive health evaluation is crucial. The guide emphasizes the importance of open communication with healthcare providers to discuss existing medical conditions. This evaluation ensures that Saxenda is prescribed with a thorough understanding of the individual's health profile.

Type 2 Diabetes and Metabolic Health

Saxenda's origins as a diabetes medication highlight its impact on metabolic health. The guide delves into the connection between Saxenda and type 2 diabetes, explaining how the medication can be especially beneficial for individuals with both weight management and diabetes control goals.

Cardiovascular Health

For individuals with cardiovascular concerns, the guide explores Saxenda's potential benefits and considerations. It discusses how weight loss can positively impact cardiovascular health and addresses any precautions or adjustments needed for individuals with specific cardiovascular conditions.

Addressing Contradictions

Contraindications and Absolute Precautions

Not everyone is a suitable candidate for Saxenda, and the guide outlines contraindications—conditions or scenarios where Saxenda is not recommended. Absolute precautions are also discussed, highlighting situations where the potential risks may outweigh the benefits, necessitating alternative weight management approaches.

History of Pancreatitis

Individuals with a history of pancreatitis require careful consideration before prescribing Saxenda. The guide explains the potential link between GLP-1 receptor agonists (of which Saxenda is one) and pancreatitis, emphasizing the importance of discussing this history with healthcare providers.

Special Considerations for Women

Pregnancy and Lactation

Saxenda's safety during pregnancy and lactation is a critical consideration. The guide provides insights into the potential risks and benefits, offering alternative strategies for weight management for individuals in these specific life stages. It encourages open dialogue with healthcare providers for personalized guidance.

3.2

This section provides a comprehensive exploration of medical conditions and considerations when considering Saxenda. By addressing the interplay between Saxenda and conditions like type 2 diabetes, cardiovascular health, and the history of pancreatitis, the guide ensures that individuals approach Saxenda with a nuanced understanding of its implications for their specific health circumstances.

Chapter 4

Getting Started with Saxenda

4.1 Consultation with Healthcare Provider
The Foundation of a Safe Weight Loss Journey
Importance of Professional Guidance
Before embarking on a Saxenda weight loss journey, a crucial first step is a consultation with a healthcare provider. The guide underscores the significance of this consultation as the foundation for a safe and effective weight management plan. A healthcare provider, often a primary care physician or an endocrinologist, plays a pivotal role in guiding individuals through the complexities of Saxenda use.

Personalized Health Assessment
During the consultation, healthcare providers conduct a personalized health assessment. This involves a detailed review of the individual's medical history, current health status, and any existing medical conditions. The guide emphasizes

the importance of transparent communication, as a thorough understanding of the individual's health profile ensures tailored recommendations.

BMI Evaluation and Eligibility

Healthcare providers assess the individual's Body Mass Index (BMI) to determine eligibility for Saxenda. The guide explains how BMI is calculated and outlines the criteria for Saxenda prescription based on specific BMI ranges. This evaluation ensures that Saxenda is recommended for individuals who stand to benefit the most from its weight loss effects.

Informed Decision-Making
Addressing Questions and Concerns

The consultation serves as a platform for individuals to ask questions and express concerns. The guide encourages readers to come prepared with a list of queries, fostering an environment where they can actively participate in decision-making. Addressing potential concerns during the consultation ensures that individuals enter into Saxenda use with a clear understanding and realistic expectations.

Understanding Risks and Benefits

Healthcare providers provide detailed information about the potential risks and benefits of Saxenda. The guide educates users on the importance of comprehending this information, empowering them to make informed decisions about their health. It stresses the collaborative nature of the healthcare provider-patient relationship in achieving successful weight loss outcomes.

Initiating Saxenda Treatment
Prescription and Dosage
Following a comprehensive consultation, healthcare providers may prescribe Saxenda. The guide outlines the typical dosage and explains the importance of adhering to the prescribed regimen. Proper understanding of the medication's administration is crucial for optimizing its effects.

Monitoring and Follow-Up
The consultation sets the stage for ongoing monitoring and follow-up appointments. Regular check-ins with the healthcare provider allow for the assessment of progress, adjustment of dosage if necessary, and addressing any emerging concerns. This iterative process ensures that Saxenda

treatment remains aligned with the individual's evolving health needs.

The consultation with a healthcare provider is a pivotal step in a Saxenda weight loss journey. By addressing the personalized health assessment, informed decision-making, and the initiation of Saxenda treatment, the guide prepares individuals for a collaborative and well-guided approach to achieving their weight loss goals.

4.2 Prescription and Dosage
Crafting a Personalized Treatment Plan
Prescribing Saxenda
Following a thorough consultation, a healthcare provider may prescribe Saxenda as part of an individual's weight management plan. The guide highlights that Saxenda is a prescription medication, reinforcing the importance of obtaining it through a licensed healthcare professional. This personalized approach ensures that the prescription aligns with the individual's specific health needs and weight loss goals.

Initial Assessment for Dosage

Upon prescribing Saxenda, healthcare providers determine the appropriate initial dosage based on factors such as the individual's overall health, response to previous weight loss efforts, and any potential contraindications. The guide emphasizes that the prescribed dosage is a critical aspect of Saxenda's effectiveness and should be followed diligently.

Understanding Saxenda Dosage

Gradual Titration for Tolerance

Saxenda is often initiated at a lower dosage to assess an individual's tolerance and minimize the risk of side effects. The guide explains the concept of gradual titration, where the dosage is increased over several weeks until the optimal therapeutic dose is reached. This cautious approach allows the body to acclimate to Saxenda, enhancing safety and tolerability.

Typical Dosage Range

The guide provides an overview of the typical dosage range for Saxenda, highlighting that individual responses may vary. While the standard starting dose is established, healthcare providers may adjust the dosage based on the individual's progress, any observed side effects, or changes in health status.

Proper Administration Techniques
Subcutaneous Injection Instructions
Saxenda is administered via subcutaneous injection, typically in the abdomen, thigh, or upper arm. The guide offers step-by-step instructions on proper injection techniques, emphasizing the importance of rotating injection sites to prevent irritation or discomfort. Clear guidance on the preparation and administration of Saxenda ensures users can integrate it seamlessly into their routine.

Adherence to Prescription
The guide stresses the importance of strict adherence to the prescribed dosage and schedule. Consistent and timely administration of Saxenda is essential for maximizing its weight loss benefits. It encourages users to communicate any challenges or concerns about the medication's administration with their healthcare providers promptly.

Monitoring and Adjustments

Regular Follow-Up Appointments

After initiating Saxenda, individuals can expect regular follow-up appointments with their healthcare providers. These appointments serve as opportunities to monitor progress, discuss any side effects or concerns, and make necessary adjustments to the dosage or treatment plan. The guide highlights the iterative nature of Saxenda treatment, emphasizing the importance of ongoing collaboration with healthcare professionals.

Prescription and Dosage provides a comprehensive understanding of the personalized nature of Saxenda treatment. By exploring the initial assessment for dosage, the gradual titration process, proper administration techniques, and the importance of adherence and monitoring, the guide equips individuals with the knowledge to navigate their Saxenda prescription confidently.

4.3 Proper Injection Techniques

Mastering the Art of Safe and Effective Saxenda Administration

Subcutaneous Injection Sites

Saxenda is administered via subcutaneous injection, where the needle is inserted into the fatty tissue just beneath the skin. The guide emphasizes that users have flexibility in choosing injection sites, typically in the abdomen, thigh, or upper arm. It provides a visual guide, detailing these areas and ensuring that users are well-informed about where to administer the injections.

Site Rotation for Comfort

To prevent irritation or discomfort, the guide underscores the importance of rotating injection sites. It explains how consistently injecting Saxenda in the same location may lead to localized reactions, and a rotational approach ensures a more comfortable experience. The guide provides a recommended schedule for site rotation, offering practical insights for users.

Preparation Steps

Proper Storage and Handling

Before delving into the injection process, the guide covers the essential steps in preparing Saxenda for administration. This includes proper storage, ensuring that the medication is kept refrigerated and protected from light. The guide also educates users on the importance of inspecting the medication for any changes in appearance before use.

Reconstitution Process
Saxenda is provided in a pen device, and users need to reconstitute the medication before the first use. The guide offers a step-by-step explanation of the reconstitution process, ensuring that users are proficient in preparing Saxenda for injection.

Checking the Pen and Dosage
Before each injection, the guide instructs users to check the pen device for any signs of damage or malfunction. It also emphasizes the importance of verifying the correct dosage before each use, promoting a vigilant approach to medication administration.

Step-by-Step Injection Guide
Cleaning the Injection Site
The guide begins the step-by-step injection process with the importance of cleaning the chosen injection site with an alcohol swab. This minimizes the risk of infection and ensures a sterile environment for the injection.

Pinch and Inject Technique
To facilitate the subcutaneous injection, the guide introduces the pinch and inject technique. It provides detailed instructions on how to pinch the skin at the injection site, creating a small fold, and then smoothly injecting Saxenda into the subcutaneous tissue.

Needle Disposal and Recap
Post-injection, the guide covers proper needle disposal and advises against recapping the needle. Safe disposal practices are essential to prevent accidental needlestick injuries.

Encouraging Open Communication
Reporting Any Discomfort or Issues
Throughout the guide, there's a strong emphasis on the importance of open communication with healthcare providers. Users are encouraged to report any discomfort, issues with injection sites, or concerns about the injection process promptly. This collaborative approach ensures that users feel supported in their Saxenda journey.

Proper Injection Techniques equips users with the knowledge and skills needed for safe and effective Saxenda administration. From understanding subcutaneous injection sites to the step-by-step injection guide and emphasizing the significance of open communication, this section ensures that individuals approach Saxenda administration with confidence and competence.

Chapter 5

Saxenda and Weight Loss

5.1 Mechanisms of Weight Loss
Unraveling Saxenda's Impact on Body Weight
Appetite Regulation
One of the primary mechanisms through which Saxenda induces weight loss is by modulating appetite. The guide delves into how Saxenda, as a synthetic GLP-1 analog, interacts with receptors in the brain responsible for appetite control. By mimicking the actions of the natural GLP-1 hormone, Saxenda reduces feelings of hunger, making it easier for individuals to adhere to a reduced-calorie diet.

Increased Satiety
Saxenda not only decreases hunger but also enhances feelings of fullness. The guide explains that this dual effect contributes to a reduction in overall food intake. Individuals find satisfaction with smaller portions, leading to a calorie deficit, a fundamental aspect of successful weight loss.

Slowed Gastric Emptying

Another critical mechanism is Saxenda's impact on gastric emptying. By slowing down the rate at which the stomach empties its contents into the intestines, Saxenda prolongs the feeling of fullness after meals. This delayed gastric emptying supports portion control and minimizes the likelihood of overeating.

Synergistic Lifestyle Changes
Integration with Diet and Exercise

The guide emphasizes that Saxenda is most effective when integrated into a comprehensive weight loss strategy. It explores how the medication complements lifestyle changes, including a reduced-calorie diet and increased physical activity. Saxenda serves as a supportive tool, enhancing the effectiveness of these lifestyle modifications.

Realistic and Sustainable Weight Loss

While Saxenda contributes to weight loss, the guide sets realistic expectations. It explains that the mechanisms of weight loss with Saxenda are gradual, promoting sustainable results. The guide encourages individuals to view weight loss as a journey, understanding that long-term success involves consistent efforts and a holistic approach.

Metabolic Impact
Regulation of Blood Glucose

Beyond its role in weight loss, Saxenda influences metabolic health. The guide outlines how Saxenda contributes to the regulation of blood glucose levels. By modulating insulin secretion in response to meals, Saxenda supports improved glucose metabolism, particularly beneficial for individuals with type 2 diabetes.

Lipid Metabolism

The guide touches on Saxenda's potential impact on lipid metabolism, explaining how weight loss and improved metabolic function may lead to positive changes in lipid profiles. This multifaceted approach underscores Saxenda's role in addressing not only weight concerns but also broader metabolic health.

Individualized Responses
Variability in Responses

The guide acknowledges that individual responses to Saxenda may vary. Factors such as genetics, lifestyle, and overall health contribute to the variability in how individuals experience weight loss with Saxenda. By recognizing this variability, the guide prepares users for a personalized journey, where adjustments may be made based on individual responses.

Mechanisms of Weight Loss provides a detailed exploration of how Saxenda influences appetite, satiety, gastric emptying, and metabolic health. By unraveling these mechanisms, the guide equips individuals with a profound understanding of how Saxenda works to support their weight loss goals in a safe and effective manner.

5.2 Clinical Studies and Efficacy
Rigorous Examination of Saxenda's Effectiveness
Overview of Clinical Studies
The guide initiates this section by providing an overview of the rigorous clinical studies conducted to assess the efficacy of Saxenda. These studies, often involving diverse participant groups, serve as the foundation for understanding how Saxenda performs in real-world scenarios.

Demonstrated Weight Loss

One of the key findings highlighted in clinical studies is Saxenda's ability to induce weight loss. The guide presents evidence of significant weight reduction among participants, emphasizing that Saxenda has consistently demonstrated effectiveness in helping individuals achieve and maintain a healthier weight.

Study Design and Methodology
Randomized Controlled Trials

The guide delves into the gold standard of clinical research — randomized controlled trials (RCTs). Saxenda's efficacy is often established through RCTs, where participants are randomly assigned to either the Saxenda group or a control group. This robust study design minimizes bias and strengthens the reliability of the findings.

Placebo-Controlled Trials

In some studies, Saxenda's efficacy is compared against a placebo. This comparison allows researchers to isolate the specific effects of Saxenda, ensuring that observed outcomes are attributable to the medication rather than external factors.

Weight Loss Trajectories

Gradual and Sustainable Weight Loss

Clinical studies consistently demonstrate that individuals using Saxenda experience gradual and sustainable weight loss. The guide emphasizes that this steady trajectory contributes to the durability of results, aligning with the goal of establishing healthy, long-term habits.

Individual Variability

While the overall trend is positive, the guide acknowledges the variability in individual responses to Saxenda. This recognition reinforces the importance of personalized treatment plans, where healthcare providers can adjust dosage or offer additional support based on an individual's unique needs.

Health Benefits Beyond Weight Loss

Improvements in Metabolic Health

Clinical studies often explore the broader health benefits associated with Saxenda use. The guide discusses findings indicating improvements in metabolic health parameters, such as better glycemic control and favorable changes in lipid profiles.

These additional benefits highlight Saxenda's potential impact on overall health beyond weight management.

Impact on Comorbidities
Saxenda's effectiveness in addressing weight-related comorbidities is highlighted in clinical studies. The guide elaborates on how improvements in weight contribute to enhanced management of conditions such as type 2 diabetes, hypertension, and dyslipidemia, reinforcing the medication's holistic impact.

Clinical Studies and Efficacy provides a thorough exploration of the robust research conducted to evaluate Saxenda's effectiveness. By examining study designs, weight loss trajectories, individual variability, and health benefits beyond weight loss, the guide equips individuals with a comprehensive understanding of the evidence supporting Saxenda as a valuable tool in achieving and maintaining a healthier weight.

5.3 Expected Results and Timelines

Setting Realistic Expectations for Saxenda Journey
Gradual and Sustainable Progress

The guide begins by establishing the principle of gradual and sustainable progress with Saxenda. It emphasizes that weight loss is a journey, not a sprint, and sets the expectation that individuals using Saxenda can anticipate steady progress over time. This approach aligns with the goal of fostering habits that contribute to long-term health.

Individual Variability

Recognizing the variability in individual responses, the guide emphasizes that expected results can differ from person to person. Factors such as genetics, lifestyle, and overall health contribute to this variability. This acknowledgment prepares users for a personalized journey, where outcomes are tailored to their unique circumstances.

Initial Weeks
Early Responses to Saxenda

The guide explores the initial weeks of Saxenda use, highlighting that some individuals may experience noticeable changes early on. This could include a reduction in appetite and an increased sense of fullness. These early responses set the stage for positive habits, reinforcing the importance of adherence to the prescribed regimen.

Gradual Weight Loss Trajectory
While early responses may be evident, the guide emphasizes that the overall weight loss trajectory with Saxenda is gradual. Users are encouraged to approach their weight loss journey with patience, understanding that sustainable results take time to manifest.

Weeks to Months
Consistent Progress Over Time
As individuals progress through weeks to months of Saxenda use, the guide communicates that consistent adherence to the medication, coupled with lifestyle changes, contributes to ongoing progress. This stage often involves a deeper integration of Saxenda into daily routines, supporting the development of sustainable habits.

Adjustments and Individualized Plans
For some individuals, healthcare providers may make adjustments to dosage or offer additional guidance based on observed responses. The guide underscores the importance of regular follow-up

appointments to facilitate these adjustments and ensure that the treatment plan remains aligned with evolving health needs.

Long-Term Outlook
Maintenance of Healthier Habits
In the long term, the guide emphasizes that Saxenda's role extends beyond weight loss to the maintenance of healthier habits. Individuals are encouraged to leverage the positive changes initiated by Saxenda to sustain a lifestyle conducive to overall well-being.

Individualized Goals
The guide recognizes that long-term success is defined by individualized goals. Whether the aim is to achieve a specific weight target or maintain improvements in metabolic health, Saxenda's role adapts to support these varied objectives.

Expected Results and Timelines provides a nuanced understanding of the Saxenda journey. By setting realistic expectations, acknowledging individual variability, and outlining the progress from the initial weeks to the long-term outlook, the guide equips individuals with the knowledge to navigate their weight loss journey with patience, commitment, and a focus on sustainable health.

Chapter 6

Nutritional Guidelines

6.1 Diet Recommendations
Synergizing Saxenda with Nutritious Choices
Importance of a Balanced Diet
The guide underscores the pivotal role of a balanced diet in conjunction with Saxenda. It emphasizes that Saxenda is most effective when integrated into a comprehensive weight loss plan that includes a nutritious and well-rounded diet. A balanced diet ensures that individuals receive essential nutrients while creating a caloric deficit for weight loss.

Caloric Intake Considerations
The guide explores the concept of caloric intake, providing insights into the importance of creating a calorie deficit for weight loss. It encourages individuals to work with healthcare providers or nutritionists to determine an appropriate caloric target based on individual factors such as age, gender, activity level, and weight loss goals.

Nutrient-Rich Food Choices

Emphasis on Whole Foods

Nutrient-rich whole foods take center stage in the guide's dietary recommendations. It advocates for the inclusion of a variety of fruits, vegetables, lean proteins, whole grains, and healthy fats. These foods not only provide essential vitamins and minerals but also contribute to a sense of fullness, aligning with Saxenda's appetite-regulating effects.

Portion Control Strategies

To enhance the effectiveness of Saxenda and support weight loss goals, the guide introduces portion control strategies. It educates individuals on mindful eating practices, emphasizing the importance of savoring each bite, recognizing hunger and fullness cues, and avoiding overconsumption.

Hydration Guidelines

Importance of Adequate Hydration

Proper hydration is highlighted in the guide's dietary recommendations. It explains how staying adequately hydrated is crucial for overall health and can also support weight loss efforts. The guide encourages individuals to prioritize water intake throughout the day and offers practical tips for maintaining hydration.

Limiting Caloric Beverages
In line with weight loss goals, the guide advises against excessive consumption of caloric beverages. It discusses the potential impact of sugary drinks on overall caloric intake and encourages the substitution of water or other low-calorie beverages.

Individualized Approach
Collaborative Decision-Making
The guide emphasizes that dietary recommendations are not one-size-fits-all and encourages collaborative decision-making between individuals and their healthcare providers or nutrition professionals. This approach ensures that dietary plans align with individual preferences, cultural considerations, and specific health needs.

Addressing Dietary Restrictions
For individuals with dietary restrictions or specific health conditions, the guide provides guidance on adapting dietary choices to meet their unique requirements. It underscores the importance of transparent communication with healthcare

providers to tailor dietary recommendations accordingly.

Sustainable Habits
Integration into Lifestyle
The guide places a strong emphasis on the sustainability of dietary habits. It encourages individuals to view dietary changes as long-term lifestyle adjustments rather than short-term fixes. This approach aligns with Saxenda's goal of supporting sustainable weight loss.

Flexibility and Enjoyment
Dietary recommendations include flexibility and enjoyment. The guide encourages individuals to find a balance that accommodates occasional indulgences and ensures a positive relationship with food. This flexibility contributes to the long-term adherence to healthier dietary choices.

Diet Recommendations provides a comprehensive guide to integrating Saxenda with a balanced and nutritious diet. By emphasizing the importance of whole foods, portion control, hydration, and individualized approaches, the guide equips individuals with the knowledge and tools to make dietary choices that complement their Saxenda weight loss journey in a sustainable and enjoyable manner.

6.2 Meal Planning

Strategic Approaches to Nourishing the Body

Purpose of Meal Planning

The guide introduces meal planning as a strategic approach to nourishing the body while supporting weight loss goals with Saxenda. It emphasizes that planning meals in advance can help individuals make informed and nutritious choices, ensuring that dietary decisions align with their overall health objectives.

Collaborative Planning

Meal planning is presented as a collaborative process between individuals and their healthcare providers or nutrition professionals. By involving professionals in the planning process, individuals can receive personalized guidance tailored to their specific dietary needs, preferences, and health conditions.

Balanced Meal Components
Inclusion of Macronutrients
The guide breaks down the components of a balanced meal, emphasizing the inclusion of macronutrients—proteins, carbohydrates, and fats. It provides insights into the role of each macronutrient in supporting overall health and how a balanced combination contributes to sustained energy and satiety.

Focus on Fiber and Nutrient Density
Meal planning encourages a focus on fiber-rich and nutrient-dense foods. These include fruits, vegetables, whole grains, and lean proteins. The guide explains that these choices not only provide essential vitamins and minerals but also contribute to a feeling of fullness, supporting weight management efforts.

Practical Meal Planning Strategies
Weekly Planning
The guide advocates for weekly meal planning as a practical strategy. Planning meals for the week allows individuals to create a well-rounded menu, make informed grocery lists, and reduce the

likelihood of spontaneous, less nutritious food choices.

Batch Cooking and Prepping

To streamline meal preparation, the guide introduces the concept of batch cooking and prepping. It explains how preparing larger quantities of certain foods in advance can save time during the week and promote consistency in adhering to a balanced diet.

Adaptability and Flexibility

Adapting to Preferences and Schedules

Meal planning is presented as an adaptable tool that can accommodate individual preferences and schedules. The guide encourages individuals to tailor their meal plans to suit their tastes, cultural considerations, and daily routines, fostering a sustainable and enjoyable approach to eating.

Flexibility for Variety

While structure is essential, the guide also emphasizes the importance of flexibility. Incorporating a variety of foods ensures a well-rounded nutritional profile and makes meal planning more enjoyable. This flexibility allows for experimentation with different recipes and cuisines.

Monitoring and Adjustments
Regular Reflection and Adjustment
Meal planning involves regular reflection on dietary choices and adjustments based on individual responses. The guide advises individuals to monitor how their bodies react to different meals and make necessary modifications to their plans. This iterative process ensures that meal planning remains a dynamic and personalized tool.

Meal Planning provides a comprehensive guide to strategic and collaborative approaches to nourishing the body while on Saxenda. By emphasizing balanced meal components, practical planning strategies, adaptability, and regular reflection, the guide equips individuals with the tools to integrate meal planning into their Saxenda weight loss journey in a sustainable and effective manner.

6.3 Combining Saxenda with Healthy Eating
Synergizing Medication with Nutrient-Rich Choices
Holistic Approach to Health

The guide positions the combination of Saxenda with healthy eating as a holistic approach to health. It emphasizes that the synergy between medication and nutrient-rich choices creates a powerful foundation for achieving and maintaining a healthier weight.

Leveraging Saxenda's Effects
Healthy eating is presented as a complementary strategy that leverages Saxenda's appetite-regulating effects. The guide explains that by making nutritious food choices, individuals can enhance the medication's impact on weight loss and overall well-being.

Nutritional Benefits of Saxenda Journey
Enhanced Nutrient Absorption
The guide explores how the Saxenda journey can positively influence nutrient absorption. By supporting weight loss and improving metabolic health, Saxenda may enhance the body's ability to absorb and utilize essential nutrients from the foods consumed.

Reduction in Empty-Calorie Intake

The combination of Saxenda with healthy eating encourages a reduction in empty-calorie intake. The guide explains that by choosing nutrient-dense foods, individuals can maximize their nutritional benefits while minimizing the consumption of foods that contribute little to overall health.

Building a Balanced Plate
Plate Method Concept
The guide introduces the plate method as a practical approach to building balanced meals. It encourages individuals to visualize their plate divided into portions for proteins, carbohydrates, vegetables, and fats. This visual aid simplifies the process of creating well-rounded and nutritious meals.

Portion Control with Saxenda
Healthy eating with Saxenda involves paying attention to portion control. The guide explains that Saxenda's appetite-regulating effects can support individuals in managing portion sizes, promoting a mindful and controlled approach to eating.

Mindful Eating Practices
Mindful Consumption of Meals

The guide advocates for mindful eating practices as part of combining Saxenda with healthy eating. It encourages individuals to savor each bite, eat without distractions, and pay attention to hunger and fullness cues. These practices contribute to a more conscious and enjoyable eating experience.

Avoidance of Emotional Eating
Healthy eating with Saxenda involves addressing emotional eating patterns. The guide provides strategies for recognizing emotional triggers, finding alternative coping mechanisms, and fostering a positive relationship with food. This approach supports a sustainable and balanced eating mindset.

Navigating Challenges
Addressing Dietary Challenges
The guide acknowledges that individuals may face challenges in adhering to healthy eating habits. It offers practical tips for overcoming obstacles such as social situations, cravings, and time constraints, ensuring that individuals can navigate these challenges while staying on track with their Saxenda journey.

Open Communication with Healthcare Providers

In cases of dietary challenges or uncertainties, the guide emphasizes the importance of open communication with healthcare providers or nutrition professionals. This collaborative approach ensures that individuals receive personalized guidance and support tailored to their unique circumstances.

Combining Saxenda with Healthy Eating provides a comprehensive guide to synergizing medication with nutrient-rich choices. By exploring the nutritional benefits of the Saxenda journey, building a balanced plate, practicing mindful eating, and addressing challenges, the guide equips individuals with the knowledge and strategies to integrate healthy eating seamlessly into their Saxenda weight loss journey.

Chapter 7

Incorporating Exercise

7.1 Importance of Physical Activity
Holistic Wellness and Weight Management
Integral Role in Weight Loss
The guide begins by highlighting the integral role of physical activity in the context of holistic wellness and weight management. It emphasizes that incorporating regular physical activity is a cornerstone of a comprehensive approach to achieving and maintaining a healthier weight.

Synergy with Saxenda
Physical activity is presented as a synergistic partner with Saxenda, enhancing the overall effectiveness of weight loss efforts. The guide explains that the combination of Saxenda and physical activity creates a powerful strategy that addresses both caloric expenditure and metabolic health.

Caloric Expenditure and Weight Loss
Creating a Caloric Deficit

One of the primary benefits of physical activity in weight management is its role in creating a caloric deficit. The guide breaks down the concept, explaining that burning more calories through activity than consumed through food contributes to weight loss. This fundamental principle aligns with the goals of Saxenda in promoting a healthy weight.

Enhancing Weight Loss Trajectory
Regular physical activity is identified as a catalyst for enhancing the weight loss trajectory. The guide underscores that combining Saxenda with exercise supports a more efficient and sustained approach to achieving weight loss goals.

Metabolic Health and Saxenda
Complementary Effects
The guide explores the complementary effects of physical activity and Saxenda on metabolic health. It explains how exercise, in conjunction with Saxenda, can contribute to improved insulin sensitivity, glucose metabolism, and lipid profiles. This dual impact enhances overall metabolic well-being.

Addressing Insulin Resistance

Physical activity is positioned as a valuable tool in addressing insulin resistance, a common concern in individuals with obesity and metabolic disorders. The guide discusses how exercise can enhance insulin sensitivity, aligning with Saxenda's multifaceted approach to metabolic health.

Mental Health and Well-Being
Mood Enhancement
Beyond its physical benefits, the guide delves into the positive impact of physical activity on mental health. It explains how exercise releases endorphins, neurotransmitters that contribute to mood enhancement and stress reduction. This mental well-being aspect aligns with Saxenda's holistic approach to overall health.

Stress Management
Physical activity is presented as an effective strategy for managing stress. The guide discusses how exercise can serve as a healthy outlet for stress, promoting emotional well-being and resilience during the weight loss journey.

Developing Sustainable Habits
Integration into Lifestyle

The guide emphasizes that the importance of physical activity extends beyond weight loss to the development of sustainable habits. It encourages individuals to view exercise as an integral part of their lifestyle, fostering a positive and enduring relationship with physical activity.

Varied Approaches to Exercise
Recognizing that individuals have diverse preferences, the guide advocates for varied approaches to exercise. It suggests exploring activities that align with personal interests, making physical activity an enjoyable and sustainable component of daily life.

Medical Considerations and Safety
Consultation with Healthcare Providers
To ensure safety, the guide underscores the importance of consulting with healthcare providers before initiating a new exercise regimen, especially in the context of Saxenda use. This collaborative approach ensures that individuals receive tailored advice based on their health status and any potential contraindications.

Gradual Progression

The guide promotes a gradual progression in physical activity, especially for individuals who may be new to exercise or have health considerations. It advises starting with activities of low intensity and gradually increasing the duration and intensity to prevent injury and enhance adherence.

7.1

The Importance of Physical Activity provides a comprehensive guide to understanding the integral role of exercise in conjunction with Saxenda for holistic wellness and weight management. By exploring its impact on caloric expenditure, metabolic health, mental well-being, sustainable habits, and safety considerations, the guide equips individuals with the knowledge and motivation to embrace physical activity as a key component of their Saxenda weight loss journey.

7.2 Suitable Exercises
Tailoring Physical Activity to Individual Preferences
Embracing Diverse Activities
The guide opens by emphasizing the importance of tailoring physical activity to individual preferences.

It encourages individuals to explore a variety of exercises, recognizing that different activities resonate with different people. By embracing diversity, the guide aims to make exercise an enjoyable and sustainable aspect of the Saxenda weight loss journey.

Considering Health and Fitness Levels

Suitable exercises are presented as those that align with an individual's health and fitness levels. The guide acknowledges that everyone has a unique starting point, and exercises should be chosen with consideration for current physical capabilities, health status, and any pre-existing conditions.

Cardiovascular Exercises

Benefits of Cardiovascular Activity

Cardiovascular exercises take center stage as suitable options for weight management with Saxenda. The guide delves into the benefits of activities such as walking, jogging, cycling, swimming, and dancing. These exercises elevate heart rate, burn calories, and contribute to the creation of a caloric deficit—a fundamental aspect of weight loss.

Gradual Progression in Cardiovascular Exercise

Recognizing that cardiovascular fitness varies among individuals, the guide emphasizes the importance of gradual progression. It advises starting with manageable durations and intensities and progressively increasing these factors as cardiovascular fitness improves. This approach ensures safety and promotes long-term adherence.

Strength Training

Role of Strength Training in Weight Management

The guide introduces strength training as a valuable component of suitable exercises for weight management. It explains how building lean muscle mass contributes to an increase in basal metabolic rate, enhancing the body's ability to burn calories even at rest.

Incorporating Resistance Training

Suitable strength training activities include weightlifting, resistance band exercises, and bodyweight exercises. The guide provides insights into incorporating these activities into a well-rounded exercise routine. It underscores the versatility of strength training, accommodating various preferences and fitness levels.

Flexibility and Balance Exercises
Enhancing Mobility and Stability
Flexibility and balance exercises are highlighted for their role in enhancing overall mobility and stability. The guide explores activities such as yoga and Pilates, emphasizing their contribution to joint flexibility, core strength, and overall body awareness.

Integrating Stretching and Balance Work
The guide offers practical tips for integrating stretching and balance work into exercise routines. These exercises not only support physical well-being but also contribute to injury prevention and an improved range of motion.

Endurance Activities
Engaging in Endurance Workouts
Endurance activities, such as hiking, cycling, or participating in group fitness classes, are presented as engaging options for suitable exercises. The guide encourages individuals to choose activities that they enjoy and that align with their endurance goals.

Social and Enjoyable Endurance Pursuits

Highlighting the social aspect of some endurance activities, the guide underscores the importance of choosing exercises that bring joy and a sense of community. Social engagement can enhance motivation and make exercise a positive and enjoyable experience.

Personalizing Exercise Routines
Tailoring Exercise Plans
Recognizing that individual preferences play a crucial role, the guide encourages individuals to personalize their exercise routines. It offers guidance on creating a well-rounded plan that combines cardiovascular exercises, strength training, flexibility work, and endurance activities based on personal interests and goals.

Consistency and Adaptability
The guide emphasizes the significance of consistency in maintaining an exercise routine. It also acknowledges the need for adaptability, allowing individuals to modify their exercise plans based on changing circumstances, preferences, or fitness levels.

Suitable Exercises provides a comprehensive guide to tailoring physical activity to individual preferences and health considerations. By exploring cardiovascular exercises, strength training, flexibility and balance activities, endurance pursuits, and the importance of personalization, the guide equips individuals with the knowledge and motivation to engage in suitable exercises that enhance their Saxenda weight loss journey in an enjoyable and sustainable manner.

7.3 Creating a Fitness Routine

Designing a Structured and Sustainable Exercise Plan

Purpose of a Fitness Routine

The guide introduces the concept of a fitness routine as a structured plan designed to promote regular physical activity. It emphasizes that creating a fitness routine serves the dual purpose of enhancing overall health and supporting weight management, especially when combined with Saxenda.

Aligning with Personal Goals

A key element in creating a fitness routine is aligning it with personal goals. The guide encourages individuals to reflect on their specific objectives, whether they include weight loss, improved cardiovascular health, strength building, or enhanced flexibility. This personalized approach ensures that the fitness routine is both meaningful and motivating.

Assessing Current Fitness Levels
Starting Point Evaluation
Creating a fitness routine begins with an assessment of current fitness levels. The guide advises individuals to honestly evaluate their endurance, strength, flexibility, and cardiovascular fitness. This self-awareness forms the foundation for tailoring the routine to individual capabilities and gradually progressing over time.

Health Considerations
Health considerations are highlighted in the assessment phase. The guide emphasizes the importance of considering any existing health conditions, past injuries, or medical recommendations. This information guides the

selection of suitable exercises and ensures that the fitness routine aligns with overall well-being.

Choosing Diverse Exercises
Comprehensive Approach
The guide advocates for a comprehensive approach to exercise selection within the fitness routine. It encourages the incorporation of diverse exercises, including cardiovascular activities, strength training, flexibility and balance exercises, and endurance pursuits. This variety ensures that the routine addresses multiple aspects of fitness.

Personal Preferences
Recognizing the role of personal preferences, the guide suggests choosing exercises that align with individual interests. Whether it's dancing, hiking, weightlifting, or yoga, the fitness routine becomes more enjoyable and sustainable when built around activities that bring satisfaction and fulfillment.

Setting Realistic Goals
SMART Goal Setting
Creating a fitness routine involves setting realistic and achievable goals. The guide introduces the SMART criteria—Specific, Measurable,

Achievable, Relevant, and Time-bound. Applying these principles ensures that goals are clear, trackable, and tailored to individual capabilities, fostering a sense of accomplishment.

Short-Term and Long-Term Goals
The guide differentiates between short-term and long-term goals within the fitness routine. Short-term goals provide milestones for regular assessment and motivation, while long-term goals contribute to the overarching vision of sustained health and fitness.

Structuring the Routine
Frequency, Duration, and Intensity
The guide provides guidance on structuring the fitness routine by determining the frequency, duration, and intensity of exercise sessions. It emphasizes the importance of gradual progression, especially for individuals new to regular physical activity. This approach ensures that the routine is challenging yet sustainable.

Balancing Different Exercise Types
Balancing different types of exercises within the routine is highlighted. The guide suggests a mix of

cardiovascular, strength, flexibility, and endurance activities to provide a holistic and well-rounded approach to fitness. This balance optimizes overall health benefits.

Incorporating Flexibility
Adaptive Approach
Recognizing that life is dynamic, the guide encourages individuals to incorporate flexibility into their fitness routines. It emphasizes an adaptive approach that allows for modifications based on changing circumstances, such as work commitments, travel, or unexpected events.

Periodic Assessments and Adjustments
The guide recommends periodic assessments of the fitness routine to evaluate progress and make necessary adjustments. This reflective practice ensures that the routine remains aligned with evolving goals, preferences, and fitness levels.

Accountability and Support
Personal and Social Accountability
Creating a fitness routine involves establishing accountability mechanisms. The guide suggests personal accountability through self-monitoring and

reflection. Additionally, social accountability, such as exercising with a friend or joining fitness classes, enhances motivation and adherence.

Seeking Professional Guidance
For individuals seeking additional support, the guide highlights the option of seeking professional guidance. This may involve working with a personal trainer, fitness instructor, or healthcare provider to tailor the fitness routine to specific needs and receive expert advice.

Creating a Fitness Routine provides a comprehensive guide to designing a structured and sustainable exercise plan. By emphasizing goal setting, assessing current fitness levels, choosing diverse exercises, setting realistic goals, structuring the routine, incorporating flexibility, and seeking accountability and support, the guide empowers individuals to embark on a fitness journey that enhances their Saxenda weight loss efforts while promoting overall health and well-being.

Chapter 8

Managing Side Effects

8.1 Common Side Effects
Understanding the Potential Effects of Saxenda
Introduction to Side Effects
The guide introduces the topic of common side effects associated with Saxenda, emphasizing the importance of understanding these effects for informed and confident medication use. It explains that while not everyone experiences side effects, being aware of potential outcomes contributes to a proactive and informed approach.

Temporary Nature of Side Effects
The guide reassures individuals that many side effects are temporary and may diminish over time as the body adjusts to Saxenda. It underscores the significance of open communication with healthcare providers to address any concerns or discomfort during the adjustment period.

Gastrointestinal Side Effects

Nausea

Nausea is identified as a common gastrointestinal side effect of Saxenda. The guide explains that individuals may experience a sensation of queasiness, especially during the initial weeks of medication use. It advises individuals to take Saxenda as prescribed and, if needed, consult with healthcare providers for guidance on managing nausea.

Vomiting

Vomiting is mentioned as a less common but possible side effect. The guide clarifies that if individuals experience persistent or severe vomiting, it is crucial to seek immediate medical attention. Healthcare providers can assess the situation and provide appropriate guidance.

Diarrhea

Diarrhea is discussed as another gastrointestinal side effect. The guide suggests maintaining hydration and consulting with healthcare providers if diarrhea persists or becomes severe. Adjustments to diet and fluid intake may be recommended to manage this side effect.

Potential Impact on Appetite

Decreased Appetite

Saxenda's impact on appetite is acknowledged, and a decreased appetite is identified as a potential side effect. The guide explains that this effect aligns with the medication's role in appetite regulation. It encourages individuals to be mindful of their dietary choices to ensure adequate nutrition while experiencing reduced hunger.

Injection Site Reactions

Redness and Irritation

The guide informs individuals about potential injection site reactions, such as redness and irritation. It explains that these reactions are usually mild and may resolve on their own. Proper injection techniques and rotation of injection sites are recommended practices to minimize discomfort.

Nodules or Lumps

The guide addresses the possibility of developing nodules or lumps at injection sites. It emphasizes the importance of informing healthcare providers if individuals notice persistent lumps or experience pain at injection sites. Healthcare providers can assess the situation and provide guidance on proper injection practices.

General Considerations
Reporting Side Effects to Healthcare Providers
The guide reinforces the importance of reporting any side effects to healthcare providers promptly. It explains that open communication allows healthcare providers to monitor individual responses to Saxenda and make necessary adjustments to dosage or provide additional support.

Differentiated Responses
Individual responses to Saxenda may vary, and the guide acknowledges that not everyone will experience the same side effects. Factors such as individual health status, lifestyle, and adherence to medication guidelines contribute to the variability in responses.

Common Side Effects provides a comprehensive understanding of the potential effects of Saxenda. By addressing gastrointestinal side effects, the impact on appetite, injection site reactions, and general considerations regarding side effect reporting, the guide equips individuals with the knowledge to navigate their Saxenda journey with awareness and confidence, ensuring a proactive and informed approach to medication use.

8.2 When to Seek Medical Attention

Recognizing Warning Signs and Taking Action

Importance of Monitoring Health

The guide underscores the importance of actively monitoring one's health while using Saxenda. It introduces the topic of when to seek medical attention, emphasizing that being aware of warning signs contributes to proactive and responsible medication use.

Clear Communication with Healthcare Providers

Maintaining clear communication with healthcare providers is highlighted as a key component of knowing when to seek medical attention. The guide encourages individuals to openly discuss any concerns or changes in their health, fostering a collaborative and supportive relationship with healthcare professionals.

Immediate Medical Attention

Severe Allergic Reactions

The guide identifies severe allergic reactions as a critical situation requiring immediate medical attention. Symptoms such as difficulty breathing, swelling of the face, lips, or tongue, and severe itching may indicate an allergic reaction. It emphasizes the importance of seeking emergency medical assistance if these symptoms occur.

Persistent or Severe Vomiting

Persistent or severe vomiting is highlighted as a situation that warrants immediate medical attention. The guide advises individuals to contact healthcare providers promptly if vomiting becomes persistent or severe. Timely intervention can help address the underlying cause and prevent complications.

Signs of Dehydration

Recognizing signs of dehydration, such as extreme thirst, dark urine, or dizziness, is emphasized. The guide advises individuals to seek medical attention if these signs are present, as dehydration can have serious health implications. Healthcare providers can assess hydration status and provide appropriate guidance.

Prompt Reporting to Healthcare Providers
Injection Site Complications
The guide discusses complications related to injection sites, such as persistent lumps, nodules, or severe pain. It advises individuals to promptly report these issues to healthcare providers. This enables healthcare professionals to assess injection techniques, provide guidance, or make adjustments to the treatment plan as needed.

Unexplained Changes in Health
Unexplained changes in health, including unexpected weight loss, unusual fatigue, or persistent changes in appetite, are highlighted as situations that warrant reporting to healthcare providers. These changes may indicate underlying health concerns that require evaluation and intervention.

Ongoing Communication with Healthcare Providers
Regular Follow-Up Appointments
The guide emphasizes the importance of attending regular follow-up appointments with healthcare providers. These appointments allow for ongoing assessment of individual responses to Saxenda and

provide opportunities to address emerging concerns or make adjustments to the treatment plan.

Transparent Communication

Transparent communication with healthcare providers is encouraged throughout the Saxenda journey. The guide advises individuals to share any changes in health, even if they may seem minor. Open communication allows healthcare providers to offer timely support and ensure that individuals feel confident and supported in their medication use.

General Guidelines for Seeking Medical Attention

Trusting Individual Instincts

Individuals are encouraged to trust their instincts and seek medical attention if they feel something is not right. The guide acknowledges that personal intuition and self-awareness play crucial roles in recognizing changes in health and making informed decisions about seeking medical assistance.

Timely Response to Concerns

Whether related to side effects, changes in health, or general discomfort, the guide stresses the importance of a timely response to concerns. Early intervention can prevent potential complications and contribute to a positive and safe Saxenda experience.

When to Seek Medical Attention provides a comprehensive guide to recognizing warning signs and taking appropriate action during Saxenda use. By highlighting situations that require immediate attention, promoting prompt reporting to healthcare providers, encouraging ongoing communication, and emphasizing the importance of individual instincts, the guide empowers individuals to navigate their Saxenda journey with vigilance and responsibility, ensuring a proactive approach to health and well-being.

8.3 Tips for Minimizing Discomfort
Proactive Strategies for a Comfortable Saxenda Experience
Introduction to Discomfort Management
The guide introduces the topic of minimizing discomfort during Saxenda use, emphasizing the proactive nature of discomfort management. It explains that by implementing certain strategies,

individuals can enhance their overall experience with the medication.

Importance of Open Communication
The guide reinforces the importance of open communication with healthcare providers regarding any discomfort experienced. Transparent dialogue allows healthcare professionals to provide tailored guidance and support based on individual responses to Saxenda.

Optimal Injection Techniques
Rotating Injection Sites
The guide emphasizes the importance of rotating injection sites to minimize discomfort. By alternating between different areas, individuals can prevent the accumulation of irritation or nodules at a specific site. Proper rotation contributes to a more comfortable injection experience.

Ensuring Correct Injection Depth
Ensuring the correct injection depth is highlighted as a key element of optimal injection techniques. The guide advises individuals to follow healthcare providers' instructions carefully, maintaining the appropriate angle and depth for injections. This

helps prevent complications and discomfort at the injection site.

Gradual Adjustment to Dosage
Starting with a Low Dosage
To minimize discomfort during the initial phases of Saxenda use, the guide suggests starting with a low dosage as prescribed by healthcare providers. This gradual approach allows the body to acclimate to the medication, potentially reducing the intensity of side effects.

Gradual Dosage Increases
For individuals experiencing discomfort with dosage increases, the guide recommends gradual adjustments. Instead of making large leaps in dosage, incremental increases give the body time to adapt, potentially minimizing side effects and discomfort associated with higher doses.

Lifestyle Considerations
Hydration Practices
The guide highlights the importance of staying adequately hydrated to support overall well-being and minimize discomfort. Proper hydration can contribute to the prevention of side effects such as

nausea and dizziness. Individuals are encouraged to maintain a consistent and sufficient fluid intake.

Consistent Meal Timing

Consistent meal timing is identified as a lifestyle consideration to minimize discomfort. The guide suggests maintaining regular meal schedules to align with Saxenda use. This practice helps regulate blood sugar levels and may contribute to reducing feelings of nausea or changes in appetite.

Supportive Measures

Using Pain Relievers

For individuals experiencing mild discomfort at injection sites, the guide suggests using over-the-counter pain relievers as directed by healthcare providers. This can help alleviate localized pain or soreness associated with injections.

Seeking Emotional Support

Emotional support is recognized as an important aspect of discomfort management. The guide encourages individuals to seek support from friends, family, or support groups, fostering a positive mindset and emotional well-being throughout the Saxenda journey.

Self-Care Practices

Prioritizing Self-Care

The guide emphasizes the importance of self-care practices to minimize overall discomfort. Adequate rest, stress management, and engaging in activities that bring joy and relaxation contribute to a holistic approach to well-being while using Saxenda.

Recognizing Personal Limits

Individuals are encouraged to recognize their personal limits and take breaks when needed. If discomfort becomes overwhelming, the guide advises individuals to consult with healthcare providers to explore potential adjustments to the Saxenda treatment plan.

Regular Follow-Up with Healthcare Providers

Scheduled Check-Ins

Regular follow-up appointments with healthcare providers are highlighted as opportunities to discuss discomfort management strategies. The guide encourages individuals to communicate openly about any challenges or concerns, allowing healthcare providers to offer guidance and adjustments as needed.

Adjustments to Treatment Plan

In cases of persistent discomfort, the guide emphasizes the importance of collaborating with healthcare providers to explore potential adjustments to the Saxenda treatment plan. This may involve modifying dosage, addressing lifestyle factors, or considering alternative approaches to enhance comfort.

Tips for Minimizing Discomfort provides a comprehensive guide to proactive strategies for a comfortable Saxenda experience. By focusing on optimal injection techniques, gradual dosage adjustments, lifestyle considerations, supportive measures, self-care practices, and regular follow-up with healthcare providers, the guide equips individuals with practical tips to enhance their overall well-being while using Saxenda.

Chapter 9

Success Stories

9.1 Real-Life Experiences
Personal Narratives of Saxenda Users
Introduction to Real-Life Experiences
The guide introduces a section dedicated to real-life experiences, aiming to provide a glimpse into the journeys of individuals who have used Saxenda. These narratives offer insights, perspectives, and diverse accounts that can resonate with readers, fostering a sense of connection and shared understanding.

Diversity of Experiences
Highlighting the diversity of experiences, the guide acknowledges that individual journeys with Saxenda can vary. Factors such as health conditions, lifestyle, and personal goals contribute to unique perspectives. Real-life experiences serve as valuable testimonials, allowing readers to relate to different aspects of the Saxenda weight loss journey.

Success Stories
Celebrating Achievements
The guide features success stories from individuals who have achieved their weight loss goals with Saxenda. These narratives celebrate the accomplishments of users, showcasing the positive impact of the medication on their lives. Success stories inspire and motivate readers, reinforcing the potential for Saxenda to contribute to meaningful weight loss transformations.

Lifestyle Changes and Sustainable Habits
Success stories often highlight not only the role of Saxenda but also the incorporation of lifestyle changes and sustainable habits. Users share how they embraced healthier eating patterns, increased physical activity, and developed positive relationships with food. These holistic approaches contribute to long-term success and well-being.

Challenges and Learnings
Honest Reflections
Real-life experiences also include narratives that candidly discuss challenges faced during the Saxenda journey. Users share their honest reflections on overcoming obstacles, navigating setbacks, and

learning from their experiences. These narratives provide a balanced perspective, acknowledging that the weight loss journey may have ups and downs.

Strategies for Overcoming Challenges
In sharing challenges, users often provide insights into the strategies they employed to overcome difficulties. Whether addressing side effects, managing lifestyle adjustments, or navigating emotional aspects of weight loss, these narratives offer practical tips and coping mechanisms that can resonate with readers facing similar challenges.

Individual Perspectives on Side Effects
Varied Responses to Medication
Real-life expericnces delve into individual perspectives on side effects, acknowledging that responses to Saxenda can differ. Users share their encounters with common side effects, such as nausea or changes in appetite, providing firsthand accounts of how they managed and adapted to these effects.

Coping Mechanisms and Support Systems
Users often discuss coping mechanisms and support systems that helped them navigate side effects.

Whether seeking guidance from healthcare providers, connecting with online communities, or relying on personal networks, these strategies contribute to a more positive and supported Saxenda experience.

Emotional and Mental Well-Being
Impact on Mental Health
Real-life experiences shed light on the emotional and mental aspects of the Saxenda journey. Users share how their weight loss efforts influenced their self-esteem, confidence, and overall well-being. These narratives highlight the interconnectedness of physical and mental health during the weight loss process.

Building a Positive Mindset
Users often discuss the importance of building a positive mindset throughout their Saxenda journey. Real-life experiences include insights into cultivating self-compassion, setting realistic goals, and maintaining a healthy relationship with one's body. These mental health considerations contribute to a holistic approach to well-being.

Decision-Making Process

Informed Choices and Shared Decision-Making
Real-life experiences explore the decision-making process that led individuals to choose Saxenda as part of their weight loss strategy. Users share their considerations, discussions with healthcare providers, and the factors that influenced their decision to incorporate Saxenda into their lives. These narratives contribute to informed choices and shared decision-making.

Collaboration with Healthcare Providers
The guide underscores the collaborative nature of decision-making, emphasizing the importance of ongoing communication with healthcare providers. Users share how their healthcare teams played a pivotal role in guiding them through the Saxenda journey, offering personalized advice, and addressing concerns.

Real-Life Experiences provides a rich tapestry of personal narratives, offering a diverse and authentic portrayal of the Saxenda weight loss journey. By featuring success stories, challenges and learnings, individual perspectives on side effects, insights into emotional and mental well-being, and reflections on the decision-making process, these real-life experiences contribute to a nuanced understanding of how Saxenda can impact lives and support individuals in achieving their weight loss goals.

9.2 Inspirational Journeys
Stories of Resilience and Transformation
Introduction to Inspirational Journeys
The guide introduces a section dedicated to inspirational journeys, aiming to showcase stories of resilience, determination, and transformation among individuals who have embarked on the Saxenda weight loss journey. These narratives inspire readers by highlighting the strength and commitment demonstrated by those who have undergone significant transformations.

Motivational Impact
The section emphasizes the motivational impact of these inspirational journeys, recognizing that stories of personal triumph can serve as powerful sources of encouragement for individuals considering or currently using Saxenda. Inspirational journeys offer a glimpse into the transformative possibilities that

the medication, coupled with lifestyle changes, can bring.

Overcoming Adversity
Triumph over Challenges
Inspirational journeys often feature individuals who have triumphed over significant challenges on their weight loss path. These challenges may include health setbacks, emotional struggles, or previous unsuccessful attempts at weight management. By sharing how they overcame adversity, these narratives instill hope and determination in readers.

Perseverance and Commitment
The guide underscores the themes of perseverance and commitment woven into inspirational journeys. Users share how they stayed dedicated to their weight loss goals, navigated setbacks, and consistently worked towards positive changes. These stories highlight the transformative power of resilience and unwavering commitment.

Lifestyle Transformations
Holistic Changes
Inspirational journeys often spotlight holistic lifestyle transformations that extend beyond weight

loss. Users share how their journeys led to improvements in overall health, increased energy levels, and enhanced well-being. These narratives showcase the broader impact of Saxenda in supporting individuals in achieving comprehensive health goals.

Positive Effects on Mental Health
Users in inspirational journeys often discuss the positive effects of their weight loss efforts on mental health. Improved self-esteem, increased confidence, and a more positive outlook on life are common themes. These aspects contribute to a holistic sense of well-being, reinforcing the interconnectedness of physical and mental health.

Motivational Strategies
Goal Setting and Tracking Progress
Inspirational journeys delve into motivational strategies employed by individuals to set and achieve their goals. Users often share insights into effective goal-setting techniques and the importance of tracking progress. These strategies empower readers with actionable tips to enhance their own motivation and goal attainment.

Celebrating Milestones

The guide highlights the significance of celebrating milestones within inspirational journeys. Users share how acknowledging and celebrating achievements, whether big or small, played a pivotal role in maintaining motivation. This practice fosters a positive and reinforcing mindset throughout the Saxenda weight loss journey.

Support Systems

Role of Supportive Networks

Inspirational journeys often underscore the role of supportive networks in achieving weight loss success. Users share how family, friends, or online communities provided encouragement, understanding, and accountability. These narratives emphasize the importance of building a strong support system for sustained motivation.

Healthcare Provider Collaboration

Collaboration with healthcare providers is a common theme in inspirational journeys. Users share how their healthcare teams played a crucial role in guiding them through the Saxenda journey, offering personalized advice, monitoring progress, and addressing any challenges. This collaborative approach contributes to a supportive and well-informed weight loss experience.

Empowerment and Self-Discovery
Empowering Changes
Inspirational journeys highlight the empowering changes experienced by individuals using Saxenda. Users share how the medication, coupled with lifestyle modifications, empowered them to take control of their health and make positive choices. These narratives reinforce the sense of agency and self-empowerment that can accompany the weight loss journey.

Discovering Personal Strength
Users often reflect on the self-discovery aspect of their journeys, acknowledging newfound strength and resilience. Inspirational narratives explore how individuals discovered inner resources, coping mechanisms, and a deeper understanding of themselves during the Saxenda weight loss process.

Inspirational Journeys provides a collection of stories that showcase the transformative power of resilience, commitment, and Saxenda use in achieving weight loss goals. By featuring narratives of overcoming adversity, holistic lifestyle transformations, motivational strategies, the role of support systems, healthcare provider collaboration, and the empowerment and self-discovery experienced by users, these inspirational journeys inspire and uplift readers on their own paths to wellness.

Chapter 10

Maintaining Weight Loss

10.1 Post-Saxenda Strategies
Transitioning Beyond Saxenda Use
Introduction to Post-Saxenda Strategies
The guide introduces a section focused on strategies for the post-Saxenda phase, recognizing that individuals may contemplate life after completing their Saxenda journey. This section aims to provide guidance on transitioning to a sustainable and healthy lifestyle, emphasizing the importance of maintaining progress and well-being.

Holistic Approach to Wellness
Highlighting a holistic approach to wellness, the section encourages individuals to consider various aspects of health beyond weight loss. Post-Saxenda strategies encompass physical activity, nutrition, mental well-being, and ongoing healthcare collaboration to ensure a comprehensive and sustained approach to health.

Maintaining Lifestyle Changes
Perpetuating Healthy Habits
Post-Saxenda strategies emphasize the importance of perpetuating the healthy habits developed during the weight loss journey. Users share insights into how they sustained positive changes in eating patterns, physical activity, and self-care practices, contributing to long-term well-being.

Building Resilience
The guide underscores the role of building resilience as individuals transition beyond Saxenda use. Post-Saxenda, users often share how they developed resilience in the face of challenges, maintained motivation, and adapted to life changes. This resilience supports ongoing commitment to a healthy lifestyle.

Continued Physical Activity
Incorporating Regular Exercise
Post-Saxenda, the guide encourages individuals to continue incorporating regular physical activity into their routines. Users share how they found joy in various exercises, whether it be walking, cycling, or engaging in fitness classes. The emphasis is on

making physical activity a sustainable and enjoyable part of daily life.

Exploring Varied Activities
To prevent monotony and sustain interest, post-Saxenda strategies include exploring a variety of physical activities. Users discuss how they diversified their exercise routines, discovering new forms of movement that align with their preferences and contribute to continued fitness.

Nutritional Considerations
Maintaining Balanced Nutrition
Post-Saxenda strategies delve into maintaining balanced nutrition beyond the medication phase. Users share how they continued making mindful food choices, emphasizing the importance of a well-rounded diet that supports overall health. This approach contributes to sustained weight management and well-being.

Mindful Eating Practices
The guide introduces mindful eating practices as part of post-Saxenda strategies. Users discuss how they cultivated awareness around their eating habits, listened to hunger and fullness cues, and embraced a

positive relationship with food. Mindful eating fosters a sustainable and mindful approach to nutrition.

Emotional Well-Being
Nurturing Mental Health
Post-Saxenda, strategies for nurturing mental health are emphasized. Users share how they prioritized self-care, managed stress, and sought support when needed. This holistic approach to emotional well-being contributes to a positive mindset and overall life satisfaction.

Coping with Changes
Acknowledging that life changes are inevitable, post-Saxenda strategies include insights into coping mechanisms. Users discuss how they navigated transitions, maintained a flexible mindset, and adapted their healthy habits to evolving circumstances. This adaptability contributes to long-term success.

Ongoing Healthcare Collaboration
Continuing Follow-Up Appointments
Post-Saxenda, the guide emphasizes the importance of continuing follow-up appointments with

healthcare providers. Users share how ongoing collaboration with healthcare teams supported their post-Saxenda journey. Regular check-ins allow for monitoring health, addressing concerns, and adjusting strategies as needed.

Seeking Professional Guidance
The section encourages individuals to seek professional guidance for post-Saxenda strategies. Whether consulting with a nutritionist, fitness trainer, or mental health professional, users discuss how tailored advice contributed to their ongoing success and well-being.

Individualized Approaches
Personalizing Post-Saxenda Strategies
Recognizing the uniqueness of each individual, post-Saxenda strategies are presented as highly personalized. Users share how they tailored their approaches to fit their preferences, health goals, and lifestyles. This individualized approach contributes to sustained motivation and success.

Adapting to Changing Needs
The guide emphasizes the importance of adapting post-Saxenda strategies to changing needs. Users

discuss how they modified their routines, goals, and habits based on evolving circumstances, ensuring that their approach to health remains relevant and achievable.

10.1

Post-Saxenda Strategies provides a comprehensive guide to transitioning beyond Saxenda use and maintaining a healthy lifestyle. By focusing on maintaining lifestyle changes, continued physical activity, nutritional considerations, emotional well-being, ongoing healthcare collaboration, and individualized approaches, these strategies empower individuals to navigate the post-Saxenda phase with resilience, adaptability, and a holistic commitment to well-being.

10.2 Long-Term Lifestyle Changes
Sustainable Practices for Lasting Well-Being
Introduction to Long-Term Lifestyle Changes
The guide introduces a section dedicated to long-term lifestyle changes, emphasizing the importance of sustainable practices for lasting well-being. This section recognizes that the Saxenda

journey is part of a broader commitment to health, encouraging individuals to adopt habits that contribute to ongoing physical, mental, and emotional well-being.

Integrating Saxenda Success into Daily Life
Highlighting the integration of Saxenda success into daily life, the section explores how individuals can carry forward the positive changes initiated during their weight loss journey. Long-term lifestyle changes encompass a holistic approach that extends beyond weight management, focusing on overall health and quality of life.

Holistic Well-Being
Embracing Holistic Health
Long-term lifestyle changes emphasize the importance of embracing holistic well-being. Users share insights into how they extended their focus beyond weight loss to include physical fitness, mental health, and emotional balance. This holistic approach contributes to a comprehensive and sustained sense of health.

Prioritizing Self-Care

The guide underscores the role of prioritizing self-care as a key element of long-term lifestyle changes. Users discuss how self-care practices, including adequate rest, stress management, and activities that bring joy, became integral to their daily routines. Prioritizing self-care fosters a positive and sustainable approach to health.

Continued Physical Activity
Making Exercise a Habit
Long-term lifestyle changes emphasize making exercise a habit rather than a temporary effort. Users share how they transformed physical activity into a consistent and enjoyable part of their daily lives. Regular exercise contributes to sustained fitness, energy levels, and overall well-being.

Incorporating Variety
To prevent monotony and sustain motivation, the section encourages incorporating a variety of physical activities into long-term lifestyle changes. Users discuss how they explored different forms of exercise, ensuring that their routines remain engaging and adaptable to changing preferences.

Balanced Nutrition

Establishing Healthy Eating Patterns

Long-term lifestyle changes delve into the establishment of healthy eating patterns. Users share how they built a foundation of balanced nutrition, making mindful and nourishing food choices a sustainable part of their lives. This approach supports ongoing well-being and weight maintenance.

Mindful Eating as a Lifestyle

The guide introduces mindful eating as a lifestyle practice within long-term changes. Users discuss how they cultivated mindfulness around eating, fostering a positive relationship with food and preventing mindless habits. Mindful eating becomes an integral part of sustaining balanced nutrition.

Emotional Resilience
Building Emotional Resilience

Long-term lifestyle changes include insights into building emotional resilience. Users discuss how they developed coping mechanisms, stress management strategies, and a positive mindset to navigate life's challenges. Emotional resilience contributes to overall mental well-being and adaptability.

Addressing Emotional Eating

Recognizing the connection between emotions and eating habits, the section explores how users addressed emotional eating as part of long-term lifestyle changes. Strategies for identifying emotional triggers, seeking support, and cultivating alternative coping mechanisms are discussed.

Ongoing Support Systems

Nurturing Supportive Networks

Long-term lifestyle changes emphasize the importance of nurturing supportive networks. Users share how family, friends, or online communities continued to play a crucial role in their health journey. Ongoing support systems contribute to motivation, accountability, and a sense of connection.

Professional Guidance

The guide underscores the value of ongoing professional guidance within long-term lifestyle changes. Users discuss how they continued to seek advice from healthcare providers, nutritionists, or fitness experts to refine their approaches and address evolving health needs.

Personalization and Adaptability

Personalized Approaches

Long-term lifestyle changes are presented as highly personalized, reflecting the uniqueness of each individual. Users share how they tailored their strategies to align with personal preferences, goals, and lifestyle, ensuring that their approach to health remains realistic and achievable.

Adaptability to Life Changes

Recognizing life's dynamic nature, the section emphasizes the adaptability of long-term lifestyle changes. Users discuss how they modified their routines in response to changing circumstances, ensuring that their health practices remain relevant and sustainable.

10.2

Long-Term Lifestyle Changes provides a comprehensive guide to adopting sustainable practices for lasting well-being. By focusing on holistic well-being, continued physical activity, balanced nutrition, emotional resilience, ongoing support systems, and the principles of personalization and adaptability, individuals are empowered to navigate the journey beyond Saxenda with a commitment to long-term health and happiness.

10.3 Preventing Weight Regain

Strategies for Sustained Weight Maintenance

Introduction to Preventing Weight Regain

The guide introduces a section dedicated to preventing weight regain, recognizing the importance of implementing strategies for sustained weight maintenance after completing the Saxenda journey. This section aims to empower individuals with practical approaches to preserve their achievements and foster a lasting sense of well-being.

Understanding the Dynamics of Weight Maintenance

Highlighting the dynamics of weight maintenance, the section acknowledges that preventing weight regain involves ongoing effort and commitment. Users share insights into how they navigated this phase, addressing challenges and implementing strategies to sustain their achievements.

Lifestyle Integration

Seamless Integration of Habits

Preventing weight regain emphasizes the seamless integration of healthy habits into daily life. Users discuss how they transformed positive changes initiated during Saxenda use into sustainable practices. This approach ensures that healthy habits become an intrinsic part of routine, reducing the likelihood of reverting to previous behaviors.

Consistency in Daily Choices

The guide underscores the importance of consistency in daily choices for preventing weight regain. Users share how they maintained a steadfast commitment to balanced nutrition, regular physical activity, and other health-promoting practices. Consistency contributes to the long-term stability of weight maintenance.

Mindful Eating Practices

Sustaining Mindful Eating

Preventing weight regain involves sustaining mindful eating practices. Users discuss how they continued to cultivate awareness around their eating habits, making conscious and intentional choices.

Mindful eating becomes a valuable tool for preventing overeating and maintaining a healthy relationship with food.

Recognizing Hunger and Fullness
The guide introduces the practice of recognizing hunger and fullness cues as part of preventing weight regain. Users share how they developed the ability to listen to their bodies, distinguishing between genuine hunger and other cues. This awareness aids in making informed and balanced food choices.

Regular Physical Activity
Long-Term Commitment to Exercise
Preventing weight regain emphasizes a long-term commitment to regular physical activity. Users share how they sustained their exercise routines, adapting to changing preferences and life circumstances. Consistent physical activity contributes to calorie expenditure and overall well-being.

Varied and Enjoyable Workouts
To maintain interest and motivation, the section encourages incorporating varied and enjoyable workouts. Users discuss how they explored different

forms of exercise, ensuring that their routines remain engaging. This approach contributes to preventing monotony and sustaining a positive attitude toward physical activity.

Establishing a Supportive Environment
Nurturing Support Systems
Preventing weight regain involves nurturing supportive environments. Users share how they continued to seek encouragement from family, friends, or online communities. Ongoing support systems play a crucial role in maintaining motivation, accountability, and a sense of connection.

Healthy Lifestyle Advocacy
The guide underscores the role of healthy lifestyle advocacy within social circles. Users discuss how they became advocates for healthy living, inspiring and influencing others in their networks. This shared commitment creates a positive environment that aligns with preventing weight regain.

Emotional Resilience
Building Resilience to Life Changes

Preventing weight regain requires building emotional resilience to navigate life changes. Users share insights into how they coped with stress, setbacks, and emotional triggers without resorting to unhealthy eating habits. Emotional resilience fosters a positive mindset and adaptability.

Strategies for Emotional Well-Being
The section explores strategies for maintaining emotional well-being as a key element of preventing weight regain. Users discuss practices such as mindfulness, stress management, and seeking professional support. Emotional well-being contributes to a balanced and sustainable approach to weight maintenance.

Ongoing Health Monitoring
Regular Check-Ins with Healthcare Providers
Preventing weight regain involves regular check-ins with healthcare providers. Users discuss how ongoing collaboration with healthcare teams supported their efforts. Regular assessments allow for monitoring health, addressing potential challenges, and adjusting strategies as needed.

Periodic Self-Assessment

The guide encourages periodic self-assessment as part of preventing weight regain. Users share how they reflected on their habits, progress, and overall well-being. Self-assessment provides valuable insights and helps individuals stay proactive in maintaining a healthy lifestyle.

Preventing Weight Regain provides a comprehensive guide to implementing strategies for sustained weight maintenance. By focusing on lifestyle integration, mindful eating practices, regular physical activity, establishing a supportive environment, building emotional resilience, and incorporating ongoing health monitoring, individuals are equipped with practical approaches to prevent weight regain and foster a lasting sense of well-being.

Chapter 11

FAQs about Saxenda

11.1 Addressing Common Queries

Providing Clarity and Guidance on Frequently Asked Questions

Introduction to Addressing Common Queries

The guide introduces a section dedicated to addressing common queries, aiming to provide clarity and guidance on frequently asked questions related to Saxenda use and the weight loss journey. This section recognizes the importance of addressing common concerns to support individuals in making informed decisions and navigating their Saxenda experience.

Accessibility and Reliability of Information

Highlighting the accessibility and reliability of information, the section emphasizes the value of addressing queries with accurate and evidence-based responses. Users are encouraged to seek reliable sources, consult healthcare providers, and use this section as a resource for common questions that may arise during their Saxenda journey.

Frequently Asked Questions

Understanding Saxenda Mechanism

Common queries often revolve around understanding the mechanism of Saxenda. The guide provides detailed explanations of how Saxenda works to promote weight loss, including its impact on appetite regulation and the central nervous system.

Safety Concerns and Side Effects

Addressing safety concerns and side effects is a key focus of the section. Users commonly inquire about the safety profile of Saxenda, potential side effects, and how to manage them. The guide provides comprehensive information, emphasizing the importance of open communication with healthcare providers.

Effectiveness and Expected Results

Queries related to the effectiveness of Saxenda and expected results are addressed in detail. The guide discusses factors influencing individual responses, the role of lifestyle changes, and realistic expectations for weight loss outcomes. Providing a balanced perspective, the section helps users set achievable goals.

Usage Guidelines and Practical Tips
Proper Injection Techniques
Common queries often include concerns about proper injection techniques. The guide offers detailed guidance on the correct way to administer Saxenda injections, including rotation of injection sites, injection depth, and other essential practices to ensure safety and effectiveness.

Dosage Adjustments and Timing
Users commonly seek information about dosage adjustments and timing. The guide provides insights into how healthcare providers determine appropriate dosages, the process of gradual adjustments, and the importance of consistent timing for optimal Saxenda use.

Combining Saxenda with Other Medications
Addressing queries about combining Saxenda with other medications is important for individuals managing multiple health conditions. The guide provides general guidance and emphasizes the

necessity of consulting healthcare providers to ensure compatibility with other medications.

Lifestyle Integration and Practical Advice

Incorporating Saxenda into Daily Life

Queries often arise about incorporating Saxenda into daily life. The guide offers practical advice on seamlessly integrating Saxenda into routines, managing injections during travel, and ensuring consistent adherence to the prescribed treatment plan.

Dietary Considerations

Common queries about dietary considerations, including meal planning and potential interactions with specific diets, are addressed. The guide provides guidance on creating a balanced meal plan, understanding nutritional needs, and making informed food choices while using Saxenda.

Exercise Recommendations

Queries related to exercise recommendations are explored in detail. The guide discusses the importance of physical activity, suitable exercises, and creating a personalized fitness routine that aligns with individual preferences and health goals.

Emotional Support and Coping Strategies
Managing Emotional Aspects of Weight Loss
Addressing queries about managing emotional aspects of weight loss is a focal point. The guide discusses the emotional impact of the Saxenda journey, coping strategies for challenges, and the importance of seeking emotional support from healthcare providers and loved ones.

Dealing with Plateaus and Setbacks
Common queries about dealing with plateaus and setbacks in the weight loss journey are acknowledged. The guide provides insights into overcoming challenges, adjusting strategies, and maintaining motivation during periods of slowed progress.

Post-Saxenda Phase and Long-Term Considerations
Post-Saxenda Strategies and Lifestyle Changes
Queries regarding post-Saxenda strategies and long-term lifestyle changes are comprehensively addressed. The guide offers guidance on transitioning beyond Saxenda use, sustaining healthy habits, and preventing weight regain through ongoing lifestyle choices.

Safety Concerns After Discontinuation

Users commonly seek information about safety concerns after discontinuing Saxenda. The guide provides guidance on monitoring health, addressing potential changes, and the importance of regular check-ins with healthcare providers.

Addressing Common Queries serves as a comprehensive resource, providing clarity and guidance on frequently asked questions related to Saxenda use and the weight loss journey. By addressing queries about Saxenda mechanisms, safety concerns, effectiveness, usage guidelines, lifestyle integration, emotional support, post-Saxenda considerations, and more, the guide empowers individuals with valuable information to enhance their understanding and confidence throughout their Saxenda journey.

11.2 Clarifying Misconceptions

Dispelling Common Myths and Providing Accurate Information

Introduction to Clarifying Misconceptions

The guide introduces a section dedicated to clarifying misconceptions, aiming to dispel common myths and provide accurate information related to Saxenda use and the weight loss journey. This section recognizes the importance of addressing misinformation to ensure individuals make informed decisions and approach their Saxenda experience with clarity.

Promoting Evidence-Based Understanding

Highlighting the importance of evidence-based understanding, the section emphasizes the need to distinguish between factual information and misconceptions. Users are encouraged to rely on reputable sources, consult healthcare providers, and use this section as a resource to correct any misunderstandings that may arise.

Misconceptions and Correct Information

Saxenda as a Magic Pill

A common misconception involves viewing Saxenda as a magic pill for instant weight loss. The guide dispels this myth by providing accurate information on Saxenda's mechanism, highlighting its role as a tool that, when combined with lifestyle changes, contributes to gradual and sustainable weight loss.

Immediate Results Expectation
Another misconception revolves around expecting immediate results with Saxenda use. The guide clarifies that weight loss is a gradual process, influenced by various factors, and realistic expectations are essential. Users are encouraged to understand the timeline for potential results and focus on sustainable progress.

Safety Concerns and Misinformation
Unsubstantiated Safety Concerns
Misinformation about safety concerns may lead to unfounded fears. The guide addresses common safety misconceptions, emphasizing Saxenda's approval by regulatory authorities and the importance of adhering to prescribed dosages under healthcare supervision for a safe experience.

Misattributing Side Effects
Users may misattribute unrelated symptoms to Saxenda use. The guide clarifies that while Saxenda

may have side effects, it is crucial to differentiate between medication-related effects and other health factors. Open communication with healthcare providers helps in addressing concerns accurately.

Diet and Exercise Misconceptions
Sole Reliance on Saxenda for Weight Loss
A misconception involves the belief that Saxenda alone is sufficient for weight loss without lifestyle changes. The guide dispels this myth, emphasizing the importance of a holistic approach that includes balanced nutrition, regular physical activity, and other healthy habits.

Excessive Eating Due to Saxenda
Misconceptions may arise about Saxenda leading to excessive eating. The guide clarifies that while Saxenda can impact appetite, it does not grant permission for unlimited food consumption. Users are encouraged to maintain mindful eating practices for effective weight management.

Misinformation About Long-Term Effects
Concerns About Long-Term Health Effects
Users may express concerns about potential long-term health effects of Saxenda. The guide

provides accurate information, citing studies and regulatory approvals, and underscores the importance of ongoing monitoring with healthcare providers for a well-informed perspective.

Misconceptions About Saxenda Dependency
A misconception involves fears of becoming dependent on Saxenda for weight management. The guide clarifies that Saxenda is a tool to support lifestyle changes, and its discontinuation requires a thoughtful transition with ongoing healthcare guidance rather than indicating dependency.

Addressing Emotional and Mental Well-Being
Misconceptions About Emotional Impact
Misconceptions may exist about Saxenda's emotional impact, such as assuming it will automatically improve mental well-being. The guide clarifies that while weight loss can positively influence mental health, addressing emotional aspects may require additional strategies and support.

Unrealistic Expectations for Emotional Changes
Users may hold unrealistic expectations regarding Saxenda's influence on emotional well-being. The

guide dispels this myth, emphasizing the multifaceted nature of emotional health and the need for comprehensive approaches beyond medication.

Clarifying Misconceptions serves as a valuable resource for dispelling common myths and providing accurate information related to Saxenda use and the weight loss journey. By addressing misconceptions about Saxenda as a magic pill, immediate results, safety concerns, diet and exercise, long-term effects, and emotional well-being, the guide empowers individuals with knowledge to approach their Saxenda experience with a clear and informed perspective.

Chapter 12

Conclusion

12.1 Recap of Key Points
Summarizing Crucial Information for Saxenda Users
Introduction to Recap of Key Points
The guide introduces a section focused on recapping key points, providing users with a concise summary of crucial information related to Saxenda use and the weight loss journey. This recap serves as a quick reference guide, allowing individuals to reinforce their understanding and navigate their Saxenda experience with clarity.

Importance of Reviewing Key Information
Highlighting the importance of reviewing key information, the section emphasizes that a thorough understanding of essential concepts is foundational for a successful Saxenda journey. Users are encouraged to revisit these key points regularly to reinforce their knowledge and make informed decisions.

Key Points Recap

Saxenda Mechanism

Saxenda operates by mimicking the hormone GLP-1 to regulate appetite and contribute to weight loss.

It is not a magic pill but a tool that, when combined with lifestyle changes, supports gradual weight loss.

Safety and Side Effects

Saxenda has been approved by regulatory authorities and is generally safe when used under healthcare supervision.

Side effects may occur, but open communication with healthcare providers helps manage and address them effectively.

Lifestyle Integration

Successful Saxenda use involves seamlessly integrating the medication into daily life.

Lifestyle changes, including balanced nutrition and regular physical activity, are crucial for optimal results.

Emotional and Mental Well-Being

Saxenda's impact on emotional well-being is multifaceted, and users should have realistic expectations.

Emotional resilience and additional support may be needed to address mental well-being aspects.

Post-Saxenda Strategies

Transitioning beyond Saxenda involves maintaining healthy habits and preventing weight regain.

Ongoing lifestyle changes, personalized approaches, and adaptability are keys to long-term success.

Addressing Common Queries

Frequently asked questions related to Saxenda mechanisms, safety concerns, and lifestyle integration have been addressed.

Seeking accurate information from reliable sources and healthcare providers is essential.

Clarifying Misconceptions

Common myths about Saxenda as a magic pill, immediate results, and long-term effects have been clarified.

Distinguishing between facts and misconceptions is crucial for an informed Saxenda experience.

The recap of key points provides users with a consolidated overview of crucial information related to Saxenda use and the weight loss journey. By summarizing key concepts, including Saxenda's mechanism, safety considerations, lifestyle integration, emotional well-being, post-Saxenda strategies, addressing common queries, and clarifying misconceptions, the guide aims to empower individuals with a comprehensive understanding for a successful and informed Saxenda journey.

12.2 Looking Ahead in Your Weight Loss Journey
Navigating Future Success and Well-Being

Introduction to Looking Ahead

The guide introduces a section dedicated to looking ahead in the weight loss journey, acknowledging that the Saxenda experience is a continuous and evolving process. This section focuses on providing insights and guidance for individuals as they progress beyond the initial stages, emphasizing sustainable practices, continued well-being, and ongoing success.

Embracing the Journey as a Continuum

Highlighting the journey as a continuum, the section encourages individuals to view weight loss and well-being as ongoing processes rather than finite endpoints. Looking ahead involves adopting a forward-thinking mindset, incorporating lessons learned, and adapting strategies for sustained success.

Long-Term Well-Being
Holistic Approach to Health
Looking ahead emphasizes a holistic approach to well-being. Beyond weight loss, individuals are encouraged to prioritize overall health, including mental, emotional, and physical aspects. Creating a balance that supports long-term well-being becomes a central focus.

Establishing Sustainable Habits
The guide underscores the importance of establishing sustainable habits for lasting success. Looking ahead involves identifying habits that can be maintained over time, ensuring that lifestyle changes contribute to ongoing health without undue stress or restriction.

Setting Realistic Goals
Beyond the Scale
Looking ahead encourages individuals to broaden their perspective on success beyond the scale. While weight loss is a significant achievement, setting goals related to improved fitness, enhanced energy levels, and overall quality of life contributes to a comprehensive sense of accomplishment.

Flexibility in Goal Setting

Recognizing the dynamic nature of health journeys, the section promotes flexibility in goal setting. Individuals are encouraged to adjust their goals as needed, allowing for adaptations to changing circumstances and personal growth throughout the weight loss journey.

Celebrating Milestones

Acknowledging Achievements

Looking ahead involves acknowledging and celebrating milestones along the way. Whether big or small, recognizing achievements reinforces positive behaviors, boosts motivation, and fosters a sense of accomplishment throughout the weight loss journey.

Cultivating a Positive Mindset

The guide emphasizes cultivating a positive mindset as an essential aspect of looking ahead. Developing resilience, practicing self-compassion, and focusing on the positive aspects of the journey contribute to a healthier and more sustainable approach to weight loss.

Continued Support Systems

Nurturing Supportive Networks

Looking ahead underscores the importance of nurturing supportive networks. Family, friends, or online communities can provide encouragement, understanding, and accountability, contributing to ongoing motivation and well-being.

Healthcare Provider Collaboration

Ongoing collaboration with healthcare providers remains crucial. Regular check-ins, open communication, and adjustments to the care plan contribute to a well-informed and supported weight loss journey.

Adapting to Life Changes
Flexibility in Strategies

Looking ahead involves recognizing and adapting to life changes. Individuals are encouraged to be flexible in their strategies, adjusting to evolving circumstances while maintaining a commitment to health and well-being.

Embracing a Growth Mindset

The guide promotes embracing a growth mindset as part of looking ahead. Viewing challenges as opportunities for learning and growth fosters resilience, adaptability, and a positive outlook throughout the weight loss journey.

Looking Ahead in Your Weight Loss Journey provides guidance for individuals as they navigate the ongoing and evolving nature of their Saxenda journey. By emphasizing long-term well-being, sustainable habits, realistic goal setting, celebrating milestones, continued support systems, adapting to life changes, and embracing a growth mindset, the guide aims to empower individuals to approach their weight loss journey with resilience, positivity, and a focus on lasting success.

www.ingramcontent.com/pod-product-compliance
Lightning Source LLC
Chambersburg PA
CBHW071832210526
45479CB00001B/94